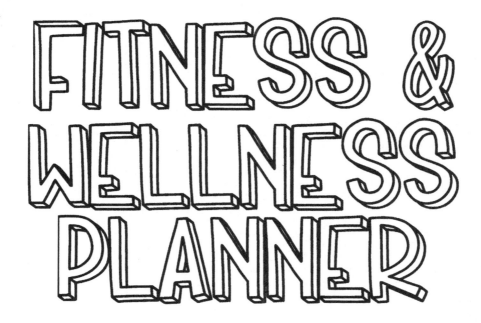

IF FOUND, PLEASE CONTACT

_____

MINDSET, THOUGHTS, FEARS, ETC.

THE PLAN

DATE: _____

STARTING IS THE HARDEST PART...

NOW		GOAL	
WEIGHT:		WEIGHT:	
CHEST:		CHEST:	
BICEP:		BICEP:	
WAIST:		WAIST:	
HIPS:		HIPS:	
THIGHS:		THIGHS:	
PANT SIZE:		PANT SIZE:	

CURRENTLY I AM...CIRCLE ONE

SLEEPING	WATER INTAKE	EXERCISE LEVEL
EH / GOOD / GREAT!	EH / GOOD / GREAT!	EH / GOOD / GREAT!

WHY DID YOU START THIS JOURNEY?...

⇒ YOU ARE WHAT YOU EAT, SO DON'T BE CHEAP, EASY OR FAKE! ⇐

WEEKLY ACTIVITIES

	TODAYS WORKOUT	SELF CARE TRACKER
SUNDAY	DATE:	SLEPT: HRS. DRINK: OZ. TODAYS MOOD:
MONDAY	DATE:	SLEPT: HRS. DRINK: OZ. TODAYS MOOD:
TUESDAY	DATE:	SLEPT: HRS. DRINK: OZ. TODAYS MOOD:
WEDNESDAY	DATE:	SLEPT: HRS. DRINK: OZ. TODAYS MOOD:
THURSDAY	DATE:	SLEPT: HRS. DRINK: OZ. TODAYS MOOD:
FRIDAY	DATE:	SLEPT: HRS. DRINK: OZ. TODAYS MOOD:
SATURDAY	DATE:	SLEPT: HRS. DRINK: OZ. TODAYS MOOD:

FUEL FOR YOUR BODY...

BREAKFAST	LUNCH	SNACKS	DINNER

PENNY FOR YOUR THOUGHTS?

WINS THIS WEEK

_____
_____
_____
_____
_____
_____
_____

3 THINGS THAT MAKE ME HAPPY

_____
_____
_____

THINGS I WANT TO IMPROVE?

_____
_____
_____
_____
_____
_____
_____

NOTES

WEEKLY ACTIVITIES

	TODAYS WORKOUT	SELF CARE TRACKER
SUNDAY	DATE:	SLEPT: HRS. DRINK: OZ. TODAYS MOOD:
MONDAY	DATE:	SLEPT: HRS. DRINK: OZ. TODAYS MOOD:
TUESDAY	DATE:	SLEPT: HRS. DRINK: OZ. TODAYS MOOD:
WEDNESDAY	DATE:	SLEPT: HRS. DRINK: OZ. TODAYS MOOD:
THURSDAY	DATE:	SLEPT: HRS. DRINK: OZ. TODAYS MOOD:
FRIDAY	DATE:	SLEPT: HRS. DRINK: OZ. TODAYS MOOD:
SATURDAY	DATE:	SLEPT: HRS. DRINK: OZ. TODAYS MOOD:

FUEL FOR YOUR BODY...

BREAKFAST	LUNCH	SNACKS	DINNER

PENNY FOR YOUR THOUGHTS?

WINS THIS WEEK

_____
_____
_____
_____
_____
_____
_____

3 THINGS THAT MAKE ME HAPPY

_____
_____
_____

THINGS I WANT TO IMPROVE?

_____
_____
_____
_____
_____
_____
_____

NOTES

WEEKLY ACTIVITIES

	TODAYS WORKOUT	SELF CARE TRACKER
SUNDAY	DATE:	SLEPT: HRS. DRINK: OZ. TODAYS MOOD:
MONDAY	DATE:	SLEPT: HRS. DRINK: OZ. TODAYS MOOD:
TUESDAY	DATE:	SLEPT: HRS. DRINK: OZ. TODAYS MOOD:
WEDNESDAY	DATE:	SLEPT: HRS. DRINK: OZ. TODAYS MOOD:
THURSDAY	DATE:	SLEPT: HRS. DRINK: OZ. TODAYS MOOD:
FRIDAY	DATE:	SLEPT: HRS. DRINK: OZ. TODAYS MOOD:
SATURDAY	DATE:	SLEPT: HRS. DRINK: OZ. TODAYS MOOD:

FUEL FOR YOUR BODY...

BREAKFAST	LUNCH	SNACKS	DINNER

PENNY FOR YOUR THOUGHTS?

WINS THIS WEEK

_____
_____
_____
_____
_____
_____
_____

3 THINGS THAT MAKE ME HAPPY

_____
_____
_____

THINGS I WANT TO IMPROVE?

_____
_____
_____
_____
_____
_____

NOTES

WEEKLY ACTIVITIES

	TODAYS WORKOUT	SELF CARE TRACKER
SUNDAY	DATE:	SLEPT: HRS. DRINK: OZ. TODAYS MOOD:
MONDAY	DATE:	SLEPT: HRS. DRINK: OZ. TODAYS MOOD:
TUESDAY	DATE:	SLEPT: HRS. DRINK: OZ. TODAYS MOOD:
WEDNESDAY	DATE:	SLEPT: HRS. DRINK: OZ. TODAYS MOOD:
THURSDAY	DATE:	SLEPT: HRS. DRINK: OZ. TODAYS MOOD:
FRIDAY	DATE:	SLEPT: HRS. DRINK: OZ. TODAYS MOOD:
SATURDAY	DATE:	SLEPT: HRS. DRINK: OZ. TODAYS MOOD:

FUEL FOR YOUR BODY...

BREAKFAST	LUNCH	SNACKS	DINNER

PENNY FOR YOUR THOUGHTS?

WINS THIS WEEK

_____
_____
_____
_____
_____
_____

3 THINGS THAT MAKE ME HAPPY

_____
_____
_____

THINGS I WANT TO IMPROVE?

_____
_____
_____
_____
_____
_____
_____

PROGRESS...

MONTH: _____

	SIZING:	CHEST:	ARMS:	WAIST:	HIPS:	THIGH:	WEIGHT:
WEEK 1							
WEEK 2							
WEEK 3							
WEEK 4							

TOTAL INCHES LOST _____

NOTES:
_____
_____
_____
_____
_____
_____
_____
_____
_____

WEEKLY ACTIVITIES

	TODAYS WORKOUT	SELF CARE TRACKER
SUNDAY	DATE:	SLEPT: HRS. DRINK: OZ. TODAYS MOOD:
MONDAY	DATE:	SLEPT: HRS. DRINK: OZ. TODAYS MOOD:
TUESDAY	DATE:	SLEPT: HRS. DRINK: OZ. TODAYS MOOD:
WEDNESDAY	DATE:	SLEPT: HRS. DRINK: OZ. TODAYS MOOD:
THURSDAY	DATE:	SLEPT: HRS. DRINK: OZ. TODAYS MOOD:
FRIDAY	DATE:	SLEPT: HRS. DRINK: OZ. TODAYS MOOD:
SATURDAY	DATE:	SLEPT: HRS. DRINK: OZ. TODAYS MOOD:

FUEL FOR YOUR BODY...

BREAKFAST	LUNCH	SNACKS	DINNER

PENNY FOR YOUR THOUGHTS?

WINS THIS WEEK

_____

_____

_____

_____

_____

_____

3 THINGS THAT MAKE ME HAPPY

_____

_____

_____

THINGS I WANT TO IMPROVE?

_____

_____

_____

_____

_____

_____

NOTES

WEEKLY ACTIVITIES

	TODAYS WORKOUT	SELF CARE TRACKER
SUNDAY	DATE:	SLEPT: HRS. DRINK: OZ. TODAYS MOOD:
MONDAY	DATE:	SLEPT: HRS. DRINK: OZ. TODAYS MOOD:
TUESDAY	DATE:	SLEPT: HRS. DRINK: OZ. TODAYS MOOD:
WEDNESDAY	DATE:	SLEPT: HRS. DRINK: OZ. TODAYS MOOD:
THURSDAY	DATE:	SLEPT: HRS. DRINK: OZ. TODAYS MOOD:
FRIDAY	DATE:	SLEPT: HRS. DRINK: OZ. TODAYS MOOD:
SATURDAY	DATE:	SLEPT: HRS. DRINK: OZ. TODAYS MOOD:

FUEL FOR YOUR BODY...

BREAKFAST	LUNCH	SNACKS	DINNER

PENNY FOR YOUR THOUGHTS?

WINS THIS WEEK

_____
_____
_____
_____
_____
_____

3 THINGS THAT MAKE ME HAPPY

_____
_____
_____

THINGS I WANT TO IMPROVE?

_____
_____
_____
_____
_____
_____
_____

NOTES

WEEKLY ACTIVITIES

	TODAYS WORKOUT	SELF CARE TRACKER
SUNDAY	DATE:	SLEPT: HRS. DRINK: OZ. TODAYS MOOD:
MONDAY	DATE:	SLEPT: HRS. DRINK: OZ. TODAYS MOOD:
TUESDAY	DATE:	SLEPT: HRS. DRINK: OZ. TODAYS MOOD:
WEDNESDAY	DATE:	SLEPT: HRS. DRINK: OZ. TODAYS MOOD:
THURSDAY	DATE:	SLEPT: HRS. DRINK: OZ. TODAYS MOOD:
FRIDAY	DATE:	SLEPT: HRS. DRINK: OZ. TODAYS MOOD:
SATURDAY	DATE:	SLEPT: HRS. DRINK: OZ. TODAYS MOOD:

FUEL FOR YOUR BODY...

BREAKFAST	LUNCH	SNACKS	DINNER

PENNY FOR YOUR THOUGHTS?

WINS THIS WEEK

_____
_____
_____
_____
_____
_____
_____

3 THINGS THAT MAKE ME HAPPY

_____
_____
_____

THINGS I WANT TO IMPROVE?

_____
_____
_____
_____
_____
_____
_____

NOTES

WEEKLY ACTIVITIES

TODAYS WORKOUT	SELF CARE TRACKER
SUNDAY DATE:	SLEPT: HRS. DRINK: OZ. TODAYS MOOD:
MONDAY DATE:	SLEPT: HRS. DRINK: OZ. TODAYS MOOD:
TUESDAY DATE:	SLEPT: HRS. DRINK: OZ. TODAYS MOOD:
WEDNESDAY DATE:	SLEPT: HRS. DRINK: OZ. TODAYS MOOD:
THURSDAY DATE:	SLEPT: HRS. DRINK: OZ. TODAYS MOOD:
FRIDAY DATE:	SLEPT: HRS. DRINK: OZ. TODAYS MOOD:
SATURDAY DATE:	SLEPT: HRS. DRINK: OZ. TODAYS MOOD:

FUEL FOR YOUR BODY...

BREAKFAST	LUNCH	SNACKS	DINNER

PENNY FOR YOUR THOUGHTS?

WINS THIS WEEK

_____
_____
_____
_____
_____
_____
_____

3 THINGS THAT MAKE ME HAPPY

_____
_____
_____

THINGS I WANT TO IMPROVE?

_____
_____
_____
_____
_____
_____

PROGRESS...

MONTH: _____

	SIZING:	CHEST:	ARMS:	WAIST:	HIPS:	THIGH:	WEIGHT:
WEEK 5							
WEEK 6							
WEEK 7							
WEEK 8							

TOTAL INCHES LOST _____

NOTES:

_____

_____

_____

_____

_____

_____

_____

_____

_____

WEEKLY ACTIVITIES

	TODAYS WORKOUT	SELF CARE TRACKER
SUNDAY	DATE:	SLEPT: HRS. DRINK: OZ. TODAYS MOOD:
MONDAY	DATE:	SLEPT: HRS. DRINK: OZ. TODAYS MOOD:
TUESDAY	DATE:	SLEPT: HRS. DRINK: OZ. TODAYS MOOD:
WEDNESDAY	DATE:	SLEPT: HRS. DRINK: OZ. TODAYS MOOD:
THURSDAY	DATE:	SLEPT: HRS. DRINK: OZ. TODAYS MOOD:
FRIDAY	DATE:	SLEPT: HRS. DRINK: OZ. TODAYS MOOD:
SATURDAY	DATE:	SLEPT: HRS. DRINK: OZ. TODAYS MOOD:

FUEL FOR YOUR BODY...

BREAKFAST	LUNCH	SNACKS	DINNER

PENNY FOR YOUR THOUGHTS?

WINS THIS WEEK

_____
_____
_____
_____
_____
_____

3 THINGS THAT MAKE ME HAPPY

_____
_____
_____

THINGS I WANT TO IMPROVE?

_____
_____
_____
_____
_____
_____
_____

NOTES

WEEKLY ACTIVITIES

TODAYS WORKOUT	SELF CARE TRACKER
SUNDAY DATE:	SLEPT: HRS. DRINK: OZ. TODAYS MOOD:
MONDAY DATE:	SLEPT: HRS. DRINK: OZ. TODAYS MOOD:
TUESDAY DATE:	SLEPT: HRS. DRINK: OZ. TODAYS MOOD:
WEDNESDAY DATE:	SLEPT: HRS. DRINK: OZ. TODAYS MOOD:
THURSDAY DATE:	SLEPT: HRS. DRINK: OZ. TODAYS MOOD:
FRIDAY DATE:	SLEPT: HRS. DRINK: OZ. TODAYS MOOD:
SATURDAY DATE:	SLEPT: HRS. DRINK: OZ. TODAYS MOOD:

FUEL FOR YOUR BODY...

BREAKFAST	LUNCH	SNACKS	DINNER

PENNY FOR YOUR THOUGHTS?

WINS THIS WEEK

_____
_____
_____
_____
_____
_____

3 THINGS THAT MAKE ME HAPPY

_____
_____
_____

THINGS I WANT TO IMPROVE?

_____
_____
_____
_____
_____
_____
_____

NOTES

WEEKLY ACTIVITIES

	TODAYS WORKOUT	SELF CARE TRACKER
SUNDAY	DATE:	SLEPT: _____ HRS. DRINK: _____ OZ. TODAYS MOOD:
MONDAY	DATE:	SLEPT: _____ HRS. DRINK: _____ OZ. TODAYS MOOD:
TUESDAY	DATE:	SLEPT: _____ HRS. DRINK: _____ OZ. TODAYS MOOD:
WEDNESDAY	DATE:	SLEPT: _____ HRS. DRINK: _____ OZ. TODAYS MOOD:
THURSDAY	DATE:	SLEPT: _____ HRS. DRINK: _____ OZ. TODAYS MOOD:
FRIDAY	DATE:	SLEPT: _____ HRS. DRINK: _____ OZ. TODAYS MOOD:
SATURDAY	DATE:	SLEPT: _____ HRS. DRINK: _____ OZ. TODAYS MOOD:

FUEL FOR YOUR BODY...

BREAKFAST	LUNCH	SNACKS	DINNER

PENNY FOR YOUR THOUGHTS?

WINS THIS WEEK
_____
_____
_____
_____
_____
_____

3 THINGS THAT MAKE ME HAPPY
_____
_____
_____

THINGS I WANT TO IMPROVE?
_____
_____
_____
_____
_____
_____

NOTES

WEEKLY ACTIVITIES

	TODAYS WORKOUT	SELF CARE TRACKER
SUNDAY	DATE:	SLEPT: HRS. DRINK: OZ. TODAYS MOOD:
MONDAY	DATE:	SLEPT: HRS. DRINK: OZ. TODAYS MOOD:
TUESDAY	DATE:	SLEPT: HRS. DRINK: OZ. TODAYS MOOD:
WEDNESDAY	DATE:	SLEPT: HRS. DRINK: OZ. TODAYS MOOD:
THURSDAY	DATE:	SLEPT: HRS. DRINK: OZ. TODAYS MOOD:
FRIDAY	DATE:	SLEPT: HRS. DRINK: OZ. TODAYS MOOD:
SATURDAY	DATE:	SLEPT: HRS. DRINK: OZ. TODAYS MOOD:

FUEL FOR YOUR BODY...

BREAKFAST	LUNCH	SNACKS	DINNER

PENNY FOR YOUR THOUGHTS?

WINS THIS WEEK

_____
_____
_____
_____
_____
_____

3 THINGS THAT MAKE ME HAPPY

_____
_____
_____

THINGS I WANT TO IMPROVE?

_____
_____
_____
_____
_____
_____

PROGRESS...

MONTH: _____

	SIZING:	CHEST:	ARMS:	WAIST:	HIPS:	THIGH:	WEIGHT:
WEEK 9							
WEEK 10							
WEEK 11							
WEEK 12							

TOTAL INCHES LOST _____

NOTES:

_____

_____

_____

_____

_____

_____

_____

_____

WEEKLY ACTIVITIES

	TODAYS WORKOUT	SELF CARE TRACKER
SUNDAY	DATE:	SLEPT: _____ HRS. DRINK: _____ OZ. TODAYS MOOD:
MONDAY	DATE:	SLEPT: _____ HRS. DRINK: _____ OZ. TODAYS MOOD:
TUESDAY	DATE:	SLEPT: _____ HRS. DRINK: _____ OZ. TODAYS MOOD:
WEDNESDAY	DATE:	SLEPT: _____ HRS. DRINK: _____ OZ. TODAYS MOOD:
THURSDAY	DATE:	SLEPT: _____ HRS. DRINK: _____ OZ. TODAYS MOOD:
FRIDAY	DATE:	SLEPT: _____ HRS. DRINK: _____ OZ. TODAYS MOOD:
SATURDAY	DATE:	SLEPT: _____ HRS. DRINK: _____ OZ. TODAYS MOOD:

FUEL FOR YOUR BODY...

BREAKFAST	LUNCH	SNACKS	DINNER

PENNY FOR YOUR THOUGHTS?

WINS THIS WEEK

_____
_____
_____
_____
_____
_____

3 THINGS THAT MAKE ME HAPPY

_____
_____
_____

THINGS I WANT TO IMPROVE?

_____
_____
_____
_____
_____
_____

NOTES

WEEKLY ACTIVITIES

	TODAYS WORKOUT	SELF CARE TRACKER
SUNDAY	DATE:	SLEPT: HRS. DRINK: OZ. TODAYS MOOD:
MONDAY	DATE:	SLEPT: HRS. DRINK: OZ. TODAYS MOOD:
TUESDAY	DATE:	SLEPT: HRS. DRINK: OZ. TODAYS MOOD:
WEDNESDAY	DATE:	SLEPT: HRS. DRINK: OZ. TODAYS MOOD:
THURSDAY	DATE:	SLEPT: HRS. DRINK: OZ. TODAYS MOOD:
FRIDAY	DATE:	SLEPT: HRS. DRINK: OZ. TODAYS MOOD:
SATURDAY	DATE:	SLEPT: HRS. DRINK: OZ. TODAYS MOOD:

FUEL FOR YOUR BODY...

BREAKFAST	LUNCH	SNACKS	DINNER

PENNY FOR YOUR THOUGHTS?

WINS THIS WEEK

_____
_____
_____
_____
_____
_____

3 THINGS THAT MAKE ME HAPPY

_____
_____
_____

THINGS I WANT TO IMPROVE?

_____
_____
_____
_____
_____
_____
_____

NOTES

WEEKLY ACTIVITIES

	TODAYS WORKOUT	SELF CARE TRACKER
SUNDAY	DATE:	SLEPT: HRS. DRINK: OZ. TODAYS MOOD:
MONDAY	DATE:	SLEPT: HRS. DRINK: OZ. TODAYS MOOD:
TUESDAY	DATE:	SLEPT: HRS. DRINK: OZ. TODAYS MOOD:
WEDNESDAY	DATE:	SLEPT: HRS. DRINK: OZ. TODAYS MOOD:
THURSDAY	DATE:	SLEPT: HRS. DRINK: OZ. TODAYS MOOD:
FRIDAY	DATE:	SLEPT: HRS. DRINK: OZ. TODAYS MOOD:
SATURDAY	DATE:	SLEPT: HRS. DRINK: OZ. TODAYS MOOD:

FUEL FOR YOUR BODY...

BREAKFAST	LUNCH	SNACKS	DINNER

PENNY FOR YOUR THOUGHTS?

WINS THIS WEEK

_____
_____
_____
_____
_____
_____
_____

3 THINGS THAT MAKE ME HAPPY

_____
_____
_____

THINGS I WANT TO IMPROVE?

_____
_____
_____
_____
_____
_____
_____

NOTES

WEEKLY ACTIVITIES

	TODAYS WORKOUT	SELF CARE TRACKER
SUNDAY	DATE:	SLEPT: HRS. DRINK: OZ. TODAYS MOOD:
MONDAY	DATE:	SLEPT: HRS. DRINK: OZ. TODAYS MOOD:
TUESDAY	DATE:	SLEPT: HRS. DRINK: OZ. TODAYS MOOD:
WEDNESDAY	DATE:	SLEPT: HRS. DRINK: OZ. TODAYS MOOD:
THURSDAY	DATE:	SLEPT: HRS. DRINK: OZ. TODAYS MOOD:
FRIDAY	DATE:	SLEPT: HRS. DRINK: OZ. TODAYS MOOD:
SATURDAY	DATE:	SLEPT: HRS. DRINK: OZ. TODAYS MOOD:

FUEL FOR YOUR BODY...

BREAKFAST	LUNCH	SNACKS	DINNER

PENNY FOR YOUR THOUGHTS?

WINS THIS WEEK
_____
_____
_____
_____
_____
_____

3 THINGS THAT MAKE ME HAPPY
_____
_____
_____

THINGS I WANT TO IMPROVE?
_____
_____
_____
_____
_____
_____

PROGRESS...

MONTH: _____

	SIZING:	CHEST:	ARMS:	WAIST:	HIPS:	THIGH:	WEIGHT:
WEEK 13							
WEEK 14							
WEEK 15							
WEEK 16							

TOTAL INCHES LOST _____

NOTES:

_____

_____

_____

_____

_____

_____

_____

_____

WEEKLY ACTIVITIES

	TODAYS WORKOUT	SELF CARE TRACKER
SUNDAY	DATE:	SLEPT: HRS. DRINK: OZ. TODAYS MOOD:
MONDAY	DATE:	SLEPT: HRS. DRINK: OZ. TODAYS MOOD:
TUESDAY	DATE:	SLEPT: HRS. DRINK: OZ. TODAYS MOOD:
WEDNESDAY	DATE:	SLEPT: HRS. DRINK: OZ. TODAYS MOOD:
THURSDAY	DATE:	SLEPT: HRS. DRINK: OZ. TODAYS MOOD:
FRIDAY	DATE:	SLEPT: HRS. DRINK: OZ. TODAYS MOOD:
SATURDAY	DATE:	SLEPT: HRS. DRINK: OZ. TODAYS MOOD:

FUEL FOR YOUR BODY...

BREAKFAST	LUNCH	SNACKS	DINNER

PENNY FOR YOUR THOUGHTS?

WINS THIS WEEK

_____
_____
_____
_____
_____
_____

3 THINGS THAT MAKE ME HAPPY

_____
_____
_____

THINGS I WANT TO IMPROVE?

_____
_____
_____
_____
_____
_____

NOTES

WEEKLY ACTIVITIES

	TODAYS WORKOUT	SELF CARE TRACKER
SUNDAY	DATE:	SLEPT: HRS. DRINK: OZ. TODAYS MOOD:
MONDAY	DATE:	SLEPT: HRS. DRINK: OZ. TODAYS MOOD:
TUESDAY	DATE:	SLEPT: HRS. DRINK: OZ. TODAYS MOOD:
WEDNESDAY	DATE:	SLEPT: HRS. DRINK: OZ. TODAYS MOOD:
THURSDAY	DATE:	SLEPT: HRS. DRINK: OZ. TODAYS MOOD:
FRIDAY	DATE:	SLEPT: HRS. DRINK: OZ. TODAYS MOOD:
SATURDAY	DATE:	SLEPT: HRS. DRINK: OZ. TODAYS MOOD:

FUEL FOR YOUR BODY...

BREAKFAST	LUNCH	SNACKS	DINNER

PENNY FOR YOUR THOUGHTS?

WINS THIS WEEK

_____
_____
_____
_____
_____
_____
_____

3 THINGS THAT MAKE ME HAPPY

_____
_____
_____

THINGS I WANT TO IMPROVE?

_____
_____
_____
_____
_____
_____
_____

NOTES

WEEKLY ACTIVITIES

	TODAYS WORKOUT	SELF CARE TRACKER
SUNDAY	DATE:	SLEPT: HRS. DRINK: OZ. TODAYS MOOD:
MONDAY	DATE:	SLEPT: HRS. DRINK: OZ. TODAYS MOOD:
TUESDAY	DATE:	SLEPT: HRS. DRINK: OZ. TODAYS MOOD:
WEDNESDAY	DATE:	SLEPT: HRS. DRINK: OZ. TODAYS MOOD:
THURSDAY	DATE:	SLEPT: HRS. DRINK: OZ. TODAYS MOOD:
FRIDAY	DATE:	SLEPT: HRS. DRINK: OZ. TODAYS MOOD:
SATURDAY	DATE:	SLEPT: HRS. DRINK: OZ. TODAYS MOOD:

FUEL FOR YOUR BODY...

BREAKFAST	LUNCH	SNACKS	DINNER

PENNY FOR YOUR THOUGHTS?

WINS THIS WEEK

_____

_____

_____

_____

_____

_____

3 THINGS THAT MAKE ME HAPPY

_____

_____

_____

THINGS I WANT TO IMPROVE?

_____

_____

_____

_____

_____

_____

_____

NOTES

WEEKLY ACTIVITIES

	TODAYS WORKOUT	SELF CARE TRACKER
SUNDAY	DATE:	SLEPT: HRS. DRINK: OZ. TODAYS MOOD:
MONDAY	DATE:	SLEPT: HRS. DRINK: OZ. TODAYS MOOD:
TUESDAY	DATE:	SLEPT: HRS. DRINK: OZ. TODAYS MOOD:
WEDNESDAY	DATE:	SLEPT: HRS. DRINK: OZ. TODAYS MOOD:
THURSDAY	DATE:	SLEPT: HRS. DRINK: OZ. TODAYS MOOD:
FRIDAY	DATE:	SLEPT: HRS. DRINK: OZ. TODAYS MOOD:
SATURDAY	DATE:	SLEPT: HRS. DRINK: OZ. TODAYS MOOD:

FUEL FOR YOUR BODY...

BREAKFAST	LUNCH	SNACKS	DINNER

PENNY FOR YOUR THOUGHTS?

WINS THIS WEEK

_____
_____
_____
_____
_____
_____
_____

3 THINGS THAT MAKE ME HAPPY

_____
_____
_____

THINGS I WANT TO IMPROVE?

_____
_____
_____
_____
_____
_____

PROGRESS...

MONTH: _____

	SIZING:	CHEST:	ARMS:	WAIST:	HIPS:	THIGH:	WEIGHT:
WEEK 17							
WEEK 18							
WEEK 19							
WEEK 20							

TOTAL INCHES LOST _____

NOTES:

_____
_____
_____
_____
_____
_____
_____
_____
_____

WEEKLY ACTIVITIES

	TODAYS WORKOUT	SELF CARE TRACKER
SUNDAY	DATE:	SLEPT: HRS. DRINK: OZ. TODAYS MOOD:
MONDAY	DATE:	SLEPT: HRS. DRINK: OZ. TODAYS MOOD:
TUESDAY	DATE:	SLEPT: HRS. DRINK: OZ. TODAYS MOOD:
WEDNESDAY	DATE:	SLEPT: HRS. DRINK: OZ. TODAYS MOOD:
THURSDAY	DATE:	SLEPT: HRS. DRINK: OZ. TODAYS MOOD:
FRIDAY	DATE:	SLEPT: HRS. DRINK: OZ. TODAYS MOOD:
SATURDAY	DATE:	SLEPT: HRS. DRINK: OZ. TODAYS MOOD:

FUEL FOR YOUR BODY...

BREAKFAST	LUNCH	SNACKS	DINNER

PENNY FOR YOUR THOUGHTS?

WINS THIS WEEK

_____
_____
_____
_____
_____
_____

3 THINGS THAT MAKE ME HAPPY

_____
_____
_____

THINGS I WANT TO IMPROVE?

_____
_____
_____
_____
_____
_____

NOTES

WEEKLY ACTIVITIES

	TODAYS WORKOUT	SELF CARE TRACKER
SUNDAY	DATE:	SLEPT: HRS. DRINK: OZ. TODAYS MOOD:
MONDAY	DATE:	SLEPT: HRS. DRINK: OZ. TODAYS MOOD:
TUESDAY	DATE:	SLEPT: HRS. DRINK: OZ. TODAYS MOOD:
WEDNESDAY	DATE:	SLEPT: HRS. DRINK: OZ. TODAYS MOOD:
THURSDAY	DATE:	SLEPT: HRS. DRINK: OZ. TODAYS MOOD:
FRIDAY	DATE:	SLEPT: HRS. DRINK: OZ. TODAYS MOOD:
SATURDAY	DATE:	SLEPT: HRS. DRINK: OZ. TODAYS MOOD:

FUEL FOR YOUR BODY...

BREAKFAST	LUNCH	SNACKS	DINNER

PENNY FOR YOUR THOUGHTS?

WINS THIS WEEK

_____
_____
_____
_____
_____
_____

3 THINGS THAT MAKE ME HAPPY

_____
_____
_____

THINGS I WANT TO IMPROVE?

_____
_____
_____
_____
_____
_____

NOTES

WEEKLY ACTIVITIES

	TODAYS WORKOUT	SELF CARE TRACKER
SUNDAY	DATE:	SLEPT: HRS. DRINK: OZ. TODAYS MOOD:
MONDAY	DATE:	SLEPT: HRS. DRINK: OZ. TODAYS MOOD:
TUESDAY	DATE:	SLEPT: HRS. DRINK: OZ. TODAYS MOOD:
WEDNESDAY	DATE:	SLEPT: HRS. DRINK: OZ. TODAYS MOOD:
THURSDAY	DATE:	SLEPT: HRS. DRINK: OZ. TODAYS MOOD:
FRIDAY	DATE:	SLEPT: HRS. DRINK: OZ. TODAYS MOOD:
SATURDAY	DATE:	SLEPT: HRS. DRINK: OZ. TODAYS MOOD:

FUEL FOR YOUR BODY...

BREAKFAST	LUNCH	SNACKS	DINNER

PENNY FOR YOUR THOUGHTS?

WINS THIS WEEK

_____

_____

_____

_____

_____

_____

3 THINGS THAT MAKE ME HAPPY

_____

_____

_____

THINGS I WANT TO IMPROVE?

_____

_____

_____

_____

_____

_____

NOTES

WEEKLY ACTIVITIES

TODAYS WORKOUT	SELF CARE TRACKER
SUNDAY DATE:	SLEPT: HRS. DRINK: OZ. TODAYS MOOD:
MONDAY DATE:	SLEPT: HRS. DRINK: OZ. TODAYS MOOD:
TUESDAY DATE:	SLEPT: HRS. DRINK: OZ. TODAYS MOOD:
WEDNESDAY DATE:	SLEPT: HRS. DRINK: OZ. TODAYS MOOD:
THURSDAY DATE:	SLEPT: HRS. DRINK: OZ. TODAYS MOOD:
FRIDAY DATE:	SLEPT: HRS. DRINK: OZ. TODAYS MOOD:
SATURDAY DATE:	SLEPT: HRS. DRINK: OZ. TODAYS MOOD:

FUEL FOR YOUR BODY...

BREAKFAST	LUNCH	SNACKS	DINNER

PENNY FOR YOUR THOUGHTS?

WINS THIS WEEK

_____
_____
_____
_____
_____
_____

3 THINGS THAT MAKE ME HAPPY

_____
_____
_____

THINGS I WANT TO IMPROVE?

_____
_____
_____
_____
_____
_____

PROGRESS...

MONTH: _____

	SIZING:	CHEST:	ARMS:	WAIST:	HIPS:	THIGH:	WEIGHT:
WEEK 21							
WEEK 22							
WEEK 23							
WEEK 24							

TOTAL INCHES LOST _____

NOTES:

_____

_____

_____

_____

_____

_____

_____

_____

_____

WEEKLY ACTIVITIES

	TODAYS WORKOUT	SELF CARE TRACKER
SUNDAY	DATE:	SLEPT: HRS. DRINK: OZ. TODAYS MOOD:
MONDAY	DATE:	SLEPT: HRS. DRINK: OZ. TODAYS MOOD:
TUESDAY	DATE:	SLEPT: HRS. DRINK: OZ. TODAYS MOOD:
WEDNESDAY	DATE:	SLEPT: HRS. DRINK: OZ. TODAYS MOOD:
THURSDAY	DATE:	SLEPT: HRS. DRINK: OZ. TODAYS MOOD:
FRIDAY	DATE:	SLEPT: HRS. DRINK: OZ. TODAYS MOOD:
SATURDAY	DATE:	SLEPT: HRS. DRINK: OZ. TODAYS MOOD:

FUEL FOR YOUR BODY...

BREAKFAST	LUNCH	SNACKS	DINNER

PENNY FOR YOUR THOUGHTS?

WINS THIS WEEK

_____
_____
_____
_____
_____
_____

3 THINGS THAT MAKE ME HAPPY

_____
_____
_____

THINGS I WANT TO IMPROVE?

_____
_____
_____
_____
_____
_____
_____

NOTES

WEEKLY ACTIVITIES

	TODAYS WORKOUT	SELF CARE TRACKER
SUNDAY	DATE:	SLEPT: HRS. DRINK: OZ. TODAYS MOOD:
MONDAY	DATE:	SLEPT: HRS. DRINK: OZ. TODAYS MOOD:
TUESDAY	DATE:	SLEPT: HRS. DRINK: OZ. TODAYS MOOD:
WEDNESDAY	DATE:	SLEPT: HRS. DRINK: OZ. TODAYS MOOD:
THURSDAY	DATE:	SLEPT: HRS. DRINK: OZ. TODAYS MOOD:
FRIDAY	DATE:	SLEPT: HRS. DRINK: OZ. TODAYS MOOD:
SATURDAY	DATE:	SLEPT: HRS. DRINK: OZ. TODAYS MOOD:

FUEL FOR YOUR BODY...

BREAKFAST	LUNCH	SNACKS	DINNER

PENNY FOR YOUR THOUGHTS?

WINS THIS WEEK
_____
_____
_____
_____
_____
_____

3 THINGS THAT MAKE ME HAPPY
_____
_____
_____

THINGS I WANT TO IMPROVE?
_____
_____
_____
_____
_____
_____
_____

NOTES

WEEKLY ACTIVITIES

	TODAYS WORKOUT	SELF CARE TRACKER
SUNDAY	DATE:	SLEPT: HRS. DRINK: OZ. TODAYS MOOD:
MONDAY	DATE:	SLEPT: HRS. DRINK: OZ. TODAYS MOOD:
TUESDAY	DATE:	SLEPT: HRS. DRINK: OZ. TODAYS MOOD:
WEDNESDAY	DATE:	SLEPT: HRS. DRINK: OZ. TODAYS MOOD:
THURSDAY	DATE:	SLEPT: HRS. DRINK: OZ. TODAYS MOOD:
FRIDAY	DATE:	SLEPT: HRS. DRINK: OZ. TODAYS MOOD:
SATURDAY	DATE:	SLEPT: HRS. DRINK: OZ. TODAYS MOOD:

FUEL FOR YOUR BODY...

BREAKFAST	LUNCH	SNACKS	DINNER

PENNY FOR YOUR THOUGHTS?

WINS THIS WEEK

_____

_____

_____

_____

_____

_____

3 THINGS THAT MAKE ME HAPPY

_____

_____

_____

THINGS I WANT TO IMPROVE?

_____

_____

_____

_____

_____

_____

NOTES

WEEKLY ACTIVITIES

TODAYS WORKOUT	SELF CARE TRACKER
SUNDAY DATE:	SLEPT: HRS. DRINK: OZ. TODAYS MOOD:
MONDAY DATE:	SLEPT: HRS. DRINK: OZ. TODAYS MOOD:
TUESDAY DATE:	SLEPT: HRS. DRINK: OZ. TODAYS MOOD:
WEDNESDAY DATE:	SLEPT: HRS. DRINK: OZ. TODAYS MOOD:
THURSDAY DATE:	SLEPT: HRS. DRINK: OZ. TODAYS MOOD:
FRIDAY DATE:	SLEPT: HRS. DRINK: OZ. TODAYS MOOD:
SATURDAY DATE:	SLEPT: HRS. DRINK: OZ. TODAYS MOOD:

FUEL FOR YOUR BODY...

BREAKFAST	LUNCH	SNACKS	DINNER

PENNY FOR YOUR THOUGHTS?

WINS THIS WEEK

_____
_____
_____
_____
_____
_____

3 THINGS THAT MAKE ME HAPPY

_____
_____
_____

THINGS I WANT TO IMPROVE?

_____
_____
_____
_____
_____
_____

PROGRESS...

MONTH: _____

	SIZING:	CHEST:	ARMS:	WAIST:	HIPS:	THIGH:	WEIGHT:
WEEK 25							
WEEK 26							
WEEK 27							
WEEK 28							

TOTAL INCHES LOST _____

NOTES:

_____

_____

_____

_____

_____

_____

_____

_____

_____

WEEKLY ACTIVITIES

	TODAYS WORKOUT	SELF CARE TRACKER
SUNDAY	DATE:	SLEPT: HRS. DRINK: OZ. TODAYS MOOD:
MONDAY	DATE:	SLEPT: HRS. DRINK: OZ. TODAYS MOOD:
TUESDAY	DATE:	SLEPT: HRS. DRINK: OZ. TODAYS MOOD:
WEDNESDAY	DATE:	SLEPT: HRS. DRINK: OZ. TODAYS MOOD:
THURSDAY	DATE:	SLEPT: HRS. DRINK: OZ. TODAYS MOOD:
FRIDAY	DATE:	SLEPT: HRS. DRINK: OZ. TODAYS MOOD:
SATURDAY	DATE:	SLEPT: HRS. DRINK: OZ. TODAYS MOOD:

FUEL FOR YOUR BODY...

BREAKFAST	LUNCH	SNACKS	DINNER

PENNY FOR YOUR THOUGHTS?

WINS THIS WEEK

_____
_____
_____
_____
_____
_____

3 THINGS THAT MAKE ME HAPPY

_____
_____
_____

THINGS I WANT TO IMPROVE?

_____
_____
_____
_____
_____
_____
_____

NOTES

WEEKLY ACTIVITIES

	TODAYS WORKOUT	SELF CARE TRACKER
SUNDAY	DATE:	SLEPT: HRS. DRINK: OZ. TODAYS MOOD:
MONDAY	DATE:	SLEPT: HRS. DRINK: OZ. TODAYS MOOD:
TUESDAY	DATE:	SLEPT: HRS. DRINK: OZ. TODAYS MOOD:
WEDNESDAY	DATE:	SLEPT: HRS. DRINK: OZ. TODAYS MOOD:
THURSDAY	DATE:	SLEPT: HRS. DRINK: OZ. TODAYS MOOD:
FRIDAY	DATE:	SLEPT: HRS. DRINK: OZ. TODAYS MOOD:
SATURDAY	DATE:	SLEPT: HRS. DRINK: OZ. TODAYS MOOD:

FUEL FOR YOUR BODY...

BREAKFAST	LUNCH	SNACKS	DINNER

PENNY FOR YOUR THOUGHTS?

WINS THIS WEEK
_____

_____
_____
_____
_____
_____
_____

3 THINGS THAT MAKE ME HAPPY
_____

_____

_____

THINGS I WANT TO IMPROVE?
_____
_____
_____
_____
_____
_____
_____
_____

NOTES

WEEKLY ACTIVITIES

	TODAYS WORKOUT	SELF CARE TRACKER
SUNDAY	DATE:	SLEPT: HRS. DRINK: OZ. TODAYS MOOD:
MONDAY	DATE:	SLEPT: HRS. DRINK: OZ. TODAYS MOOD:
TUESDAY	DATE:	SLEPT: HRS. DRINK: OZ. TODAYS MOOD:
WEDNESDAY	DATE:	SLEPT: HRS. DRINK: OZ. TODAYS MOOD:
THURSDAY	DATE:	SLEPT: HRS. DRINK: OZ. TODAYS MOOD:
FRIDAY	DATE:	SLEPT: HRS. DRINK: OZ. TODAYS MOOD:
SATURDAY	DATE:	SLEPT: HRS. DRINK: OZ. TODAYS MOOD:

FUEL FOR YOUR BODY...

BREAKFAST	LUNCH	SNACKS	DINNER

PENNY FOR YOUR THOUGHTS?

WINS THIS WEEK

_____
_____
_____
_____
_____
_____

3 THINGS THAT MAKE ME HAPPY

_____
_____
_____

THINGS I WANT TO IMPROVE?

_____
_____
_____
_____
_____
_____
_____

NOTES

WEEKLY ACTIVITIES

	TODAYS WORKOUT	SELF CARE TRACKER
SUNDAY	DATE:	SLEPT: HRS. DRINK: OZ. TODAYS MOOD:
MONDAY	DATE:	SLEPT: HRS. DRINK: OZ. TODAYS MOOD:
TUESDAY	DATE:	SLEPT: HRS. DRINK: OZ. TODAYS MOOD:
WEDNESDAY	DATE:	SLEPT: HRS. DRINK: OZ. TODAYS MOOD:
THURSDAY	DATE:	SLEPT: HRS. DRINK: OZ. TODAYS MOOD:
FRIDAY	DATE:	SLEPT: HRS. DRINK: OZ. TODAYS MOOD:
SATURDAY	DATE:	SLEPT: HRS. DRINK: OZ. TODAYS MOOD:

FUEL FOR YOUR BODY...

BREAKFAST	LUNCH	SNACKS	DINNER

PENNY FOR YOUR THOUGHTS?

WINS THIS WEEK

_____
_____
_____
_____
_____
_____

3 THINGS THAT MAKE ME HAPPY

_____
_____
_____

THINGS I WANT TO IMPROVE?

_____
_____
_____
_____
_____
_____

PROGRESS...

MONTH: _____

	SIZING:	CHEST:	ARMS:	WAIST:	HIPS:	THIGH:	WEIGHT:
WEEK 29							
WEEK 30							
WEEK 31							
WEEK 32							

TOTAL INCHES LOST _____

NOTES:

_____

_____

_____

_____

_____

_____

_____

_____

WEEKLY ACTIVITIES

	TODAYS WORKOUT	SELF CARE TRACKER
SUNDAY	DATE:	SLEPT: HRS. DRINK: OZ. TODAYS MOOD:
MONDAY	DATE:	SLEPT: HRS. DRINK: OZ. TODAYS MOOD:
TUESDAY	DATE:	SLEPT: HRS. DRINK: OZ. TODAYS MOOD:
WEDNESDAY	DATE:	SLEPT: HRS. DRINK: OZ. TODAYS MOOD:
THURSDAY	DATE:	SLEPT: HRS. DRINK: OZ. TODAYS MOOD:
FRIDAY	DATE:	SLEPT: HRS. DRINK: OZ. TODAYS MOOD:
SATURDAY	DATE:	SLEPT: HRS. DRINK: OZ. TODAYS MOOD:

FUEL FOR YOUR BODY...

BREAKFAST	LUNCH	SNACKS	DINNER

PENNY FOR YOUR THOUGHTS?

WINS THIS WEEK

_____
_____
_____
_____
_____
_____

3 THINGS THAT MAKE ME HAPPY

_____
_____
_____

THINGS I WANT TO IMPROVE?

_____
_____
_____
_____
_____
_____

NOTES

WEEKLY ACTIVITIES

	TODAYS WORKOUT	SELF CARE TRACKER
SUNDAY	DATE:	SLEPT: HRS. DRINK: OZ. TODAYS MOOD:
MONDAY	DATE:	SLEPT: HRS. DRINK: OZ. TODAYS MOOD:
TUESDAY	DATE:	SLEPT: HRS. DRINK: OZ. TODAYS MOOD:
WEDNESDAY	DATE:	SLEPT: HRS. DRINK: OZ. TODAYS MOOD:
THURSDAY	DATE:	SLEPT: HRS. DRINK: OZ. TODAYS MOOD:
FRIDAY	DATE:	SLEPT: HRS. DRINK: OZ. TODAYS MOOD:
SATURDAY	DATE:	SLEPT: HRS. DRINK: OZ. TODAYS MOOD:

FUEL FOR YOUR BODY...

BREAKFAST	LUNCH	SNACKS	DINNER

PENNY FOR YOUR THOUGHTS?

WINS THIS WEEK

_____
_____
_____
_____
_____
_____

3 THINGS THAT MAKE ME HAPPY

_____
_____
_____

THINGS I WANT TO IMPROVE?

_____
_____
_____
_____
_____
_____
_____

NOTES

WEEKLY ACTIVITIES

	TODAYS WORKOUT	SELF CARE TRACKER
SUNDAY	DATE:	SLEPT: HRS. DRINK: OZ. TODAYS MOOD:
MONDAY	DATE:	SLEPT: HRS. DRINK: OZ. TODAYS MOOD:
TUESDAY	DATE:	SLEPT: HRS. DRINK: OZ. TODAYS MOOD:
WEDNESDAY	DATE:	SLEPT: HRS. DRINK: OZ. TODAYS MOOD:
THURSDAY	DATE:	SLEPT: HRS. DRINK: OZ. TODAYS MOOD:
FRIDAY	DATE:	SLEPT: HRS. DRINK: OZ. TODAYS MOOD:
SATURDAY	DATE:	SLEPT: HRS. DRINK: OZ. TODAYS MOOD:

FUEL FOR YOUR BODY...

BREAKFAST	LUNCH	SNACKS	DINNER

PENNY FOR YOUR THOUGHTS?

WINS THIS WEEK

_____
_____
_____
_____
_____
_____

3 THINGS THAT MAKE ME HAPPY

_____
_____
_____

THINGS I WANT TO IMPROVE?

_____
_____
_____
_____
_____
_____

NOTES

WEEKLY ACTIVITIES

	TODAYS WORKOUT	SELF CARE TRACKER
SUNDAY	DATE:	SLEPT: ___ HRS. DRINK: ___ OZ. TODAYS MOOD:
MONDAY	DATE:	SLEPT: ___ HRS. DRINK: ___ OZ. TODAYS MOOD:
TUESDAY	DATE:	SLEPT: ___ HRS. DRINK: ___ OZ. TODAYS MOOD:
WEDNESDAY	DATE:	SLEPT: ___ HRS. DRINK: ___ OZ. TODAYS MOOD:
THURSDAY	DATE:	SLEPT: ___ HRS. DRINK: ___ OZ. TODAYS MOOD:
FRIDAY	DATE:	SLEPT: ___ HRS. DRINK: ___ OZ. TODAYS MOOD:
SATURDAY	DATE:	SLEPT: ___ HRS. DRINK: ___ OZ. TODAYS MOOD:

FUEL FOR YOUR BODY...

BREAKFAST	LUNCH	SNACKS	DINNER

PENNY FOR YOUR THOUGHTS?

WINS THIS WEEK

_____
_____
_____
_____
_____
_____
_____

3 THINGS THAT MAKE ME HAPPY

_____
_____
_____

THINGS I WANT TO IMPROVE?

_____
_____
_____
_____
_____
_____
_____

PROGRESS...

MONTH: _____

	SIZING:	CHEST:	ARMS:	WAIST:	HIPS:	THIGH:	WEIGHT:
WEEK 33							
WEEK 34							
WEEK 35							
WEEK 36							

TOTAL INCHES LOST _____

NOTES:

_____
_____
_____
_____
_____
_____
_____
_____
_____

WEEKLY ACTIVITIES

	TODAYS WORKOUT	SELF CARE TRACKER
SUNDAY	DATE:	SLEPT: HRS. DRINK: OZ. TODAYS MOOD:
MONDAY	DATE:	SLEPT: HRS. DRINK: OZ. TODAYS MOOD:
TUESDAY	DATE:	SLEPT: HRS. DRINK: OZ. TODAYS MOOD:
WEDNESDAY	DATE:	SLEPT: HRS. DRINK: OZ. TODAYS MOOD:
THURSDAY	DATE:	SLEPT: HRS. DRINK: OZ. TODAYS MOOD:
FRIDAY	DATE:	SLEPT: HRS. DRINK: OZ. TODAYS MOOD:
SATURDAY	DATE:	SLEPT: HRS. DRINK: OZ. TODAYS MOOD:

FUEL FOR YOUR BODY...

BREAKFAST	LUNCH	SNACKS	DINNER

PENNY FOR YOUR THOUGHTS?

WINS THIS WEEK

_____
_____
_____
_____
_____
_____

3 THINGS THAT MAKE ME HAPPY

_____
_____
_____

THINGS I WANT TO IMPROVE?

_____
_____
_____
_____
_____
_____

NOTES

WEEKLY ACTIVITIES

	TODAYS WORKOUT	SELF CARE TRACKER
SUNDAY	DATE:	SLEPT: HRS. DRINK: OZ. TODAYS MOOD:
MONDAY	DATE:	SLEPT: HRS. DRINK: OZ. TODAYS MOOD:
TUESDAY	DATE:	SLEPT: HRS. DRINK: OZ. TODAYS MOOD:
WEDNESDAY	DATE:	SLEPT: HRS. DRINK: OZ. TODAYS MOOD:
THURSDAY	DATE:	SLEPT: HRS. DRINK: OZ. TODAYS MOOD:
FRIDAY	DATE:	SLEPT: HRS. DRINK: OZ. TODAYS MOOD:
SATURDAY	DATE:	SLEPT: HRS. DRINK: OZ. TODAYS MOOD:

FUEL FOR YOUR BODY...

BREAKFAST	LUNCH	SNACKS	DINNER

PENNY FOR YOUR THOUGHTS?

WINS THIS WEEK

_____

_____

_____

_____

_____

_____

3 THINGS THAT MAKE ME HAPPY

_____

_____

_____

THINGS I WANT TO IMPROVE?

_____

_____

_____

_____

_____

_____

NOTES

WEEKLY ACTIVITIES

	TODAYS WORKOUT	SELF CARE TRACKER
SUNDAY	DATE:	SLEPT: HRS. DRINK: OZ. TODAYS MOOD:
MONDAY	DATE:	SLEPT: HRS. DRINK: OZ. TODAYS MOOD:
TUESDAY	DATE:	SLEPT: HRS. DRINK: OZ. TODAYS MOOD:
WEDNESDAY	DATE:	SLEPT: HRS. DRINK: OZ. TODAYS MOOD:
THURSDAY	DATE:	SLEPT: HRS. DRINK: OZ. TODAYS MOOD:
FRIDAY	DATE:	SLEPT: HRS. DRINK: OZ. TODAYS MOOD:
SATURDAY	DATE:	SLEPT: HRS. DRINK: OZ. TODAYS MOOD:

FUEL FOR YOUR BODY...

BREAKFAST	LUNCH	SNACKS	DINNER

PENNY FOR YOUR THOUGHTS?

WINS THIS WEEK

_____
_____
_____
_____
_____
_____
_____

3 THINGS THAT MAKE ME HAPPY

_____
_____
_____

THINGS I WANT TO IMPROVE?

_____
_____
_____
_____
_____
_____

NOTES

WEEKLY ACTIVITIES

	TODAYS WORKOUT	SELF CARE TRACKER
SUNDAY	DATE:	SLEPT: HRS. DRINK: OZ. TODAYS MOOD:
MONDAY	DATE:	SLEPT: HRS. DRINK: OZ. TODAYS MOOD:
TUESDAY	DATE:	SLEPT: HRS. DRINK: OZ. TODAYS MOOD:
WEDNESDAY	DATE:	SLEPT: HRS. DRINK: OZ. TODAYS MOOD:
THURSDAY	DATE:	SLEPT: HRS. DRINK: OZ. TODAYS MOOD:
FRIDAY	DATE:	SLEPT: HRS. DRINK: OZ. TODAYS MOOD:
SATURDAY	DATE:	SLEPT: HRS. DRINK: OZ. TODAYS MOOD:

FUEL FOR YOUR BODY...

BREAKFAST	LUNCH	SNACKS	DINNER

PENNY FOR YOUR THOUGHTS?

WINS THIS WEEK
_____
_____
_____
_____
_____

3 THINGS THAT MAKE ME HAPPY
_____
_____
_____

THINGS I WANT TO IMPROVE?
_____
_____
_____
_____
_____
_____

PROGRESS...

MONTH: _____

	SIZING:	CHEST:	ARMS:	WAIST:	HIPS:	THIGH:	WEIGHT:
WEEK 37							
WEEK 38							
WEEK 39							
WEEK 40							

TOTAL INCHES LOST _____

NOTES:

_____
_____
_____
_____
_____
_____
_____
_____

WEEKLY ACTIVITIES

	TODAYS WORKOUT	SELF CARE TRACKER
SUNDAY	DATE:	SLEPT: HRS. DRINK: OZ. TODAYS MOOD:
MONDAY	DATE:	SLEPT: HRS. DRINK: OZ. TODAYS MOOD:
TUESDAY	DATE:	SLEPT: HRS. DRINK: OZ. TODAYS MOOD:
WEDNESDAY	DATE:	SLEPT: HRS. DRINK: OZ. TODAYS MOOD:
THURSDAY	DATE:	SLEPT: HRS. DRINK: OZ. TODAYS MOOD:
FRIDAY	DATE:	SLEPT: HRS. DRINK: OZ. TODAYS MOOD:
SATURDAY	DATE:	SLEPT: HRS. DRINK: OZ. TODAYS MOOD:

FUEL FOR YOUR BODY...

BREAKFAST	LUNCH	SNACKS	DINNER

PENNY FOR YOUR THOUGHTS?

WINS THIS WEEK

_____
_____
_____
_____
_____
_____

3 THINGS THAT MAKE ME HAPPY

_____
_____
_____

THINGS I WANT TO IMPROVE?

_____
_____
_____
_____
_____
_____

NOTES

WEEKLY ACTIVITIES

	TODAYS WORKOUT	SELF CARE TRACKER
SUNDAY	DATE:	SLEPT: HRS. DRINK: OZ. TODAYS MOOD:
MONDAY	DATE:	SLEPT: HRS. DRINK: OZ. TODAYS MOOD:
TUESDAY	DATE:	SLEPT: HRS. DRINK: OZ. TODAYS MOOD:
WEDNESDAY	DATE:	SLEPT: HRS. DRINK: OZ. TODAYS MOOD:
THURSDAY	DATE:	SLEPT: HRS. DRINK: OZ. TODAYS MOOD:
FRIDAY	DATE:	SLEPT: HRS. DRINK: OZ. TODAYS MOOD:
SATURDAY	DATE:	SLEPT: HRS. DRINK: OZ. TODAYS MOOD:

FUEL FOR YOUR BODY...

BREAKFAST	LUNCH	SNACKS	DINNER

PENNY FOR YOUR THOUGHTS?

WINS THIS WEEK

_____
_____
_____
_____
_____
_____
_____

3 THINGS THAT MAKE ME HAPPY

_____
_____
_____

THINGS I WANT TO IMPROVE?

_____
_____
_____
_____
_____
_____
_____

NOTES

WEEKLY ACTIVITIES

	TODAYS WORKOUT	SELF CARE TRACKER
SUNDAY	DATE:	SLEPT: HRS. DRINK: OZ. TODAYS MOOD:
MONDAY	DATE:	SLEPT: HRS. DRINK: OZ. TODAYS MOOD:
TUESDAY	DATE:	SLEPT: HRS. DRINK: OZ. TODAYS MOOD:
WEDNESDAY	DATE:	SLEPT: HRS. DRINK: OZ. TODAYS MOOD:
THURSDAY	DATE:	SLEPT: HRS. DRINK: OZ. TODAYS MOOD:
FRIDAY	DATE:	SLEPT: HRS. DRINK: OZ. TODAYS MOOD:
SATURDAY	DATE:	SLEPT: HRS. DRINK: OZ. TODAYS MOOD:

FUEL FOR YOUR BODY...

BREAKFAST	LUNCH	SNACKS	DINNER

PENNY FOR YOUR THOUGHTS?

WINS THIS WEEK

_____

_____

_____

_____

_____

_____

3 THINGS THAT MAKE ME HAPPY

_____

_____

_____

THINGS I WANT TO IMPROVE?

_____

_____

_____

_____

_____

_____

NOTES

WEEKLY ACTIVITIES

	TODAYS WORKOUT	SELF CARE TRACKER
SUNDAY	DATE:	SLEPT: HRS. DRINK: OZ. TODAYS MOOD:
MONDAY	DATE:	SLEPT: HRS. DRINK: OZ. TODAYS MOOD:
TUESDAY	DATE:	SLEPT: HRS. DRINK: OZ. TODAYS MOOD:
WEDNESDAY	DATE:	SLEPT: HRS. DRINK: OZ. TODAYS MOOD:
THURSDAY	DATE:	SLEPT: HRS. DRINK: OZ. TODAYS MOOD:
FRIDAY	DATE:	SLEPT: HRS. DRINK: OZ. TODAYS MOOD:
SATURDAY	DATE:	SLEPT: HRS. DRINK: OZ. TODAYS MOOD:

FUEL FOR YOUR BODY...

BREAKFAST	LUNCH	SNACKS	DINNER

PENNY FOR YOUR THOUGHTS?

WINS THIS WEEK

_____
_____
_____
_____
_____
_____

3 THINGS THAT MAKE ME HAPPY

_____
_____
_____

THINGS I WANT TO IMPROVE?

_____
_____
_____
_____
_____
_____
_____

PROGRESS...

MONTH: _____

	SIZING:	CHEST:	ARMS:	WAIST:	HIPS:	THIGH:	WEIGHT:
WEEK 41							
WEEK 42							
WEEK 43							
WEEK 44							

TOTAL INCHES LOST _____

NOTES:

_____

_____

_____

_____

_____

_____

_____

_____

WEEKLY ACTIVITIES

TODAYS WORKOUT	SELF CARE TRACKER
SUNDAY DATE:	SLEPT: HRS. DRINK: OZ. TODAYS MOOD:
MONDAY DATE:	SLEPT: HRS. DRINK: OZ. TODAYS MOOD:
TUESDAY DATE:	SLEPT: HRS. DRINK: OZ. TODAYS MOOD:
WEDNESDAY DATE:	SLEPT: HRS. DRINK: OZ. TODAYS MOOD:
THURSDAY DATE:	SLEPT: HRS. DRINK: OZ. TODAYS MOOD:
FRIDAY DATE:	SLEPT: HRS. DRINK: OZ. TODAYS MOOD:
SATURDAY DATE:	SLEPT: HRS. DRINK: OZ. TODAYS MOOD:

FUEL FOR YOUR BODY...

BREAKFAST	LUNCH	SNACKS	DINNER

PENNY FOR YOUR THOUGHTS?

WINS THIS WEEK

_____
_____
_____
_____
_____
_____

3 THINGS THAT MAKE ME HAPPY

_____
_____
_____

THINGS I WANT TO IMPROVE?

_____
_____
_____
_____
_____
_____

NOTES

WEEKLY ACTIVITIES

	TODAYS WORKOUT	SELF CARE TRACKER
SUNDAY	DATE:	SLEPT: HRS. DRINK: OZ. TODAYS MOOD:
MONDAY	DATE:	SLEPT: HRS. DRINK: OZ. TODAYS MOOD:
TUESDAY	DATE:	SLEPT: HRS. DRINK: OZ. TODAYS MOOD:
WEDNESDAY	DATE:	SLEPT: HRS. DRINK: OZ. TODAYS MOOD:
THURSDAY	DATE:	SLEPT: HRS. DRINK: OZ. TODAYS MOOD:
FRIDAY	DATE:	SLEPT: HRS. DRINK: OZ. TODAYS MOOD:
SATURDAY	DATE:	SLEPT: HRS. DRINK: OZ. TODAYS MOOD:

FUEL FOR YOUR BODY...

BREAKFAST	LUNCH	SNACKS	DINNER

PENNY FOR YOUR THOUGHTS?

WINS THIS WEEK
_____
_____
_____
_____
_____
_____

3 THINGS THAT MAKE ME HAPPY
_____
_____
_____

THINGS I WANT TO IMPROVE?
_____
_____
_____
_____
_____
_____

NOTES

WEEKLY ACTIVITIES

	TODAYS WORKOUT	SELF CARE TRACKER
SUNDAY	DATE:	SLEPT: HRS. DRINK: OZ. TODAYS MOOD:
MONDAY	DATE:	SLEPT: HRS. DRINK: OZ. TODAYS MOOD:
TUESDAY	DATE:	SLEPT: HRS. DRINK: OZ. TODAYS MOOD:
WEDNESDAY	DATE:	SLEPT: HRS. DRINK: OZ. TODAYS MOOD:
THURSDAY	DATE:	SLEPT: HRS. DRINK: OZ. TODAYS MOOD:
FRIDAY	DATE:	SLEPT: HRS. DRINK: OZ. TODAYS MOOD:
SATURDAY	DATE:	SLEPT: HRS. DRINK: OZ. TODAYS MOOD:

FUEL FOR YOUR BODY...

BREAKFAST	LUNCH	SNACKS	DINNER

PENNY FOR YOUR THOUGHTS?

WINS THIS WEEK
_____
_____
_____
_____
_____
_____

3 THINGS THAT MAKE ME HAPPY
_____
_____
_____

THINGS I WANT TO IMPROVE?
_____
_____
_____
_____
_____
_____

NOTES

WEEKLY ACTIVITIES

	TODAYS WORKOUT	SELF CARE TRACKER
SUNDAY	DATE:	SLEPT: HRS. DRINK: OZ. TODAYS MOOD:
MONDAY	DATE:	SLEPT: HRS. DRINK: OZ. TODAYS MOOD:
TUESDAY	DATE:	SLEPT: HRS. DRINK: OZ. TODAYS MOOD:
WEDNESDAY	DATE:	SLEPT: HRS. DRINK: OZ. TODAYS MOOD:
THURSDAY	DATE:	SLEPT: HRS. DRINK: OZ. TODAYS MOOD:
FRIDAY	DATE:	SLEPT: HRS. DRINK: OZ. TODAYS MOOD:
SATURDAY	DATE:	SLEPT: HRS. DRINK: OZ. TODAYS MOOD:

FUEL FOR YOUR BODY...

BREAKFAST	LUNCH	SNACKS	DINNER

PENNY FOR YOUR THOUGHTS?

WINS THIS WEEK

_____
_____
_____
_____
_____
_____

3 THINGS THAT MAKE ME HAPPY

_____
_____
_____

THINGS I WANT TO IMPROVE?

_____
_____
_____
_____
_____
_____

PROGRESS...

MONTH: _____

	SIZING:	CHEST:	ARMS:	WAIST:	HIPS:	THIGH:	WEIGHT:
WEEK 45							
WEEK 46							
WEEK 47							
WEEK 48							

TOTAL INCHES LOST _____

NOTES:
_____
_____
_____
_____
_____
_____
_____
_____
_____

WEEKLY ACTIVITIES

	TODAYS WORKOUT	SELF CARE TRACKER
SUNDAY	DATE:	SLEPT: HRS. DRINK: OZ. TODAYS MOOD:
MONDAY	DATE:	SLEPT: HRS. DRINK: OZ. TODAYS MOOD:
TUESDAY	DATE:	SLEPT: HRS. DRINK: OZ. TODAYS MOOD:
WEDNESDAY	DATE:	SLEPT: HRS. DRINK: OZ. TODAYS MOOD:
THURSDAY	DATE:	SLEPT: HRS. DRINK: OZ. TODAYS MOOD:
FRIDAY	DATE:	SLEPT: HRS. DRINK: OZ. TODAYS MOOD:
SATURDAY	DATE:	SLEPT: HRS. DRINK: OZ. TODAYS MOOD:

FUEL FOR YOUR BODY...

BREAKFAST	LUNCH	SNACKS	DINNER

PENNY FOR YOUR THOUGHTS?

WINS THIS WEEK

_____
_____
_____
_____
_____
_____
_____

3 THINGS THAT MAKE ME HAPPY

_____
_____
_____

THINGS I WANT TO IMPROVE?

_____
_____
_____
_____
_____
_____
_____

NOTES

WEEKLY ACTIVITIES

	TODAYS WORKOUT	SELF CARE TRACKER
SUNDAY	DATE:	SLEPT: _____ HRS. DRINK: _____ OZ. TODAYS MOOD:
MONDAY	DATE:	SLEPT: _____ HRS. DRINK: _____ OZ. TODAYS MOOD:
TUESDAY	DATE:	SLEPT: _____ HRS. DRINK: _____ OZ. TODAYS MOOD:
WEDNESDAY	DATE:	SLEPT: _____ HRS. DRINK: _____ OZ. TODAYS MOOD:
THURSDAY	DATE:	SLEPT: _____ HRS. DRINK: _____ OZ. TODAYS MOOD:
FRIDAY	DATE:	SLEPT: _____ HRS. DRINK: _____ OZ. TODAYS MOOD:
SATURDAY	DATE:	SLEPT: _____ HRS. DRINK: _____ OZ. TODAYS MOOD:

FUEL FOR YOUR BODY...

BREAKFAST	LUNCH	SNACKS	DINNER

PENNY FOR YOUR THOUGHTS?

WINS THIS WEEK

_____
_____
_____
_____
_____
_____

3 THINGS THAT MAKE ME HAPPY

_____
_____
_____

THINGS I WANT TO IMPROVE?

_____
_____
_____
_____
_____
_____
_____

NOTES

WEEKLY ACTIVITIES

	TODAYS WORKOUT	SELF CARE TRACKER
SUNDAY	DATE:	SLEPT: HRS. DRINK: OZ. TODAYS MOOD:
MONDAY	DATE:	SLEPT: HRS. DRINK: OZ. TODAYS MOOD:
TUESDAY	DATE:	SLEPT: HRS. DRINK: OZ. TODAYS MOOD:
WEDNESDAY	DATE:	SLEPT: HRS. DRINK: OZ. TODAYS MOOD:
THURSDAY	DATE:	SLEPT: HRS. DRINK: OZ. TODAYS MOOD:
FRIDAY	DATE:	SLEPT: HRS. DRINK: OZ. TODAYS MOOD:
SATURDAY	DATE:	SLEPT: HRS. DRINK: OZ. TODAYS MOOD:

FUEL FOR YOUR BODY...

BREAKFAST	LUNCH	SNACKS	DINNER

PENNY FOR YOUR THOUGHTS?

WINS THIS WEEK

_____
_____
_____
_____
_____
_____

3 THINGS THAT MAKE ME HAPPY

_____
_____
_____

THINGS I WANT TO IMPROVE?

_____
_____
_____
_____
_____
_____

NOTES

WEEKLY ACTIVITIES

	TODAYS WORKOUT	SELF CARE TRACKER
SUNDAY	DATE:	SLEPT: HRS. DRINK: OZ. TODAYS MOOD:
MONDAY	DATE:	SLEPT: HRS. DRINK: OZ. TODAYS MOOD:
TUESDAY	DATE:	SLEPT: HRS. DRINK: OZ. TODAYS MOOD:
WEDNESDAY	DATE:	SLEPT: HRS. DRINK: OZ. TODAYS MOOD:
THURSDAY	DATE:	SLEPT: HRS. DRINK: OZ. TODAYS MOOD:
FRIDAY	DATE:	SLEPT: HRS. DRINK: OZ. TODAYS MOOD:
SATURDAY	DATE:	SLEPT: HRS. DRINK: OZ. TODAYS MOOD:

FUEL FOR YOUR BODY...

BREAKFAST	LUNCH	SNACKS	DINNER

PENNY FOR YOUR THOUGHTS?

WINS THIS WEEK

_____
_____
_____
_____
_____
_____

3 THINGS THAT MAKE ME HAPPY

_____
_____
_____

THINGS I WANT TO IMPROVE?

_____
_____
_____
_____
_____
_____

PROGRESS...

MONTH: _____

	SIZING:	CHEST:	ARMS:	WAIST:	HIPS:	THIGH:	WEIGHT:
WEEK 49							
WEEK 50							
WEEK 51							
WEEK 58							

TOTAL INCHES LOST _____

NOTES:

_____

_____

_____

_____

_____

_____

_____

_____

THE RESULT

DATE: _____

RESULTS COME OVER TIME NOT OVER NIGHT...

GOAL

WEIGHT:

CHEST:

BICEP:

WAIST:

HIPS:

THIGHS:

PANT SIZE:

ACTUAL

WEIGHT:

CHEST:

BICEP:

WAIST:

HIPS:

THIGHS:

PANT SIZE:

CURRENTLY I AM...CIRCLE ONE

SLEEPING	WATER INTAKE	EXERCISE LEVEL
EH / GOOD / GREAT!	EH / GOOD / GREAT!	EH / GOOD / GREAT!

WHAT DID YOU LEARN ON THIS JOURNEY?

 THE BODY ACHIEVES WHAT THE MIND BELIEVES

FINAL THOUGHTS...

FINAL THOUGHTS...

Made in the USA
Coppell, TX
24 April 2021